Pretty Girl Pretty Divine Beauty

Ashley M. Black

Table of Contents

~ She is clothed with strength and dignity; she can laugh at the days to come. ~

Proverbs 31:25

The Uniqueness of this book

This book puts into words which are backed up by scripture; divine womanhood, who women are in God through Jesus Christ, fashion, skin care, hair care, friend girls, women as warriors, mental health, physical health, and men. The book is unique because it describes the lifestyle and standard of a woman of God. This book is meant to provide golden nuggets on divine womanhood. I desire to attract attention to Psalm 139:14 Amplified Bible which declares, "I will give thanks and praise to You, for I am fearfully and wonderfully made; Wonderful are Your works, And my soul knows it very well." As women of God we are called to obey the Word of God and look to the scripture for instruction on conduct and standards to adhere to. I also would like to call attention to 1 Timothy 2:9 Amplified Bible which declares, "Likewise, *I want* women to adorn themselves modestly *and* appropriately and discreetly in proper clothing". Oh, what a delight it is to live in harmony and oneness with God. Women are divine as beautiful creations of God.

Summary

This book is addressing divine womanhood, who women are in God through Jesus Christ, fashion, skin care, hair care, friend girls, mental health, women as warriors, physical health, and men. This book is also a tool for the young woman who may be a babe in Christ; written for the purpose of jump-starting her faith in Christ. Of course, these topics are just as much of a concern to the Godly woman as it is to women as a whole. God's standard for the modern-day woman of God is timeless. God's standards for the modern-day woman is still alive and relevant. God our Heavenly Father, Jesus our Lord, and Holy Spirit who is God's Spirit are one and is still active in regards to earthbound activity. Women of God are still called and expected to live their lives at a higher standard. Divine womanhood and regal womanhood go hand in hand. Women are called and expected to live a lifestyle pleasing to the Father. Women of God are called to be divine and regal regardless of their social status, economic status, race, and nationality. Divine, in regards to this book, simply means Godlike, beautiful, delightful, and excellent in physical form as well as in character. Regal, in regards to this book, simply means dignified and excellent in physical form as well as in character. The world prides itself on running after superficial status and things. However, women of God are instructed to seek first the kingdom of God and his righteousness; and all these things shall be given unto them as well. The woman of God's top priority is to first seek the kingdom of God. The woman of God's ultimate goal is to become one with God through our Lord Jesus Christ and to be led of His Holy Spirit. May the words of our Lord and Savior Jesus Christ continue to ring out in to our natural as well as our spiritual ears, "If ye love me, keep my commandments".

Knowing Who You Are in God
*You are a woman of God's Creation

You are divinely beautiful. Genesis 1:27-28 King James Version declares, "So God created man in his own image, in the image of God created he him; male and female created he them. And God blessed them,". God created male and female and blessed them. You, woman of God, are made in the image and the likeness of God. When He sees you, He sees His workmanship. You are marvelous in His eyes. You were bought with the blood of His beloved son, Jesus Christ. You are fearfully and wonderfully made and your soul should know that right well.

Once you have confessed with your mouth that Jesus is Lord, and believe in your heart that God raised Him from the dead, you shall be saved. You are then a part of the family and kingdom of God. Your Heavenly Father is now responsible for you. Of course, there is work on your part to do to develop an ongoing fellowship with the Lord: devotion, prayer, study, worship, and participating in advancing the kingdom. However, be assured that your Heavenly Father takes full delight in being responsible for you and your family. Your soul, spirit, and body are His to take care of, lead, and govern. He has you in the palm of His hand and no one can pluck you out of His safe and secure hands. John

10:28-29 King James Version declares, "And I (Jesus Christ) give unto them eternal life; and they shall never perish, neither shall any man pluck them out of my hand. My Father, which gave them to me, is greater than all; and no man is able to pluck them out of my Father's hand". Your responsibility is to stay close to God (our Heavenly Father), study the Word of God, pray, and to stay in a posture of worship. God's Holy Spirit will always be with you to counsel you, comfort you, guide you, fellowship with you, and to be a friend. He knows that you love Him when you obey Him. The Father, the Son, and Holy Spirit will make their abode with you. John 14:23 New International Version declares, "Jesus replied, Anyone who loves me will obey my teaching. My Father will love them, and we will come to them and make our home with them".

Your Heavenly Father says that you are beautiful. You are divinely beautiful. Declare it, decree it, and believe it. However, humble yourselves before the Lord, and he will lift you up (James 4:10 NIV). The reward of the humble is promotion by God.

~ Her price *is* far above rubies. ~

Proverbs 31:30

Fashion
*Modesty is Best

Fashion can be used to express your inner self, your mindset, your creative style, and your standards whether high or low. Unfortunately, women are judged and stereotyped by how they look and what they wear. It is also true that the presence of God's Spirit (Holy Spirit) or the lack thereof can be seen by the choice of fashion worn. When your inner self matches or does not match your outer appearance it is a mirror and or manifestation that is either in agreement or conflicting with your inner self. As a woman of God, God's Spirit (Holy Spirit) will govern your choices. Women who have given their lives to Jesus Christ are to fashion themselves with modesty. Modesty is a behavior, manner, or appearance intended to avoid indecency. Women of God are to avoid indecent behavior on all levels including their choice of fashion.

Your beauty and God's glory seen on your life will attract people regardless of what you wear. However, you are responsible for presenting yourself as honorable while reflecting reverence, holiness, and piety in regards to your relationship with God. Modesty is not intended to attract improper attention, is not revealing, is not vain, is not to degrade self and others, and it's not to offend others. Women of God chose comfort and modesty over trends especially trends and fashions that God wouldn't be pleased with. Revealing clothing is not Godly. Revealing and flashing body parts such as breast, buttocks, and thighs are not Godly behaviors. A great undergarment foundation (support bras, shapewear, and slips) will improve your posture as well as give you confidence. Appropriately sized clothing gives you comfort as well as confidence. Clothing that is too tight or too loose is oftentimes unsightly and ungodly.

Women of God are not intentionally intending to entice men with sensual attire. A Godly woman is to have a public and private lifestyle of high standards and morals always. Your private struggles should be discussed with God through earnest prayer and supplication. The God of your salvation knows how to deliver you from any secret besetting sin. God loves you and is perfecting everything that concerns you. You are divinely beautiful. Declare it, decree it, and believe it. However, humble yourselves before the Lord, and he will lift you up (James 4:10 NIV). The reward of the humble is promotion by God.

~ Likewise, *I want* women to adorn themselves modestly *and* appropriately and discreetly in proper clothing, ~

1 Timothy 2:9

Skin Care
*Self Care is a Must

Skin care is a great part of self-care and maintenance of a woman's femininity. Taking care of your skin especially the skin on your face is so important. Your face is one of the first things people see when looking at and noticing you. Your skin may not always be blemish-free. However, well kept, bright, and clean skin is a must. A bright face with a bright smile makes all the difference. A bright face and a bright smile display confidence and it's also welcoming. A bright face and a bright smile make others feel good about you. A great personal skin care routine or regimen (a systemic plan or treatment) is worth the investment.

Invest in yourself a skin care regimen consisting of a cleanser, day moisturizer, night moisturizer, eye cream, and exfoliator or deep cleansing mask. Of course, you can customize your skin care regimen to your liking. Ponder on Queen Esther's purification process found in Esther 2 verse 12 which says, "she had to complete twelve months of beauty treatments prescribed for the women, six months with oil of myrrh and six with perfumes and cosmetics" (NIV). This is an example of a great at home spa treatment. Skin care, hair, and nails are a part of self-care maintenance. A woman of God must be well kept at all times. Great skin care makes you feel so good inside and out. Our Heavenly Father delights in you and is pleased when you take care of your temple (body) inside and out. He knows that you are divinely beautiful. Declare it, decree it, and believe it. However, humble yourselves before the Lord, and he will lift you up (James 4:10 NIV). The reward of the humble is promotion by God.

~ I beseech you therefore, brethren, by the mercies of God, that ye present your bodies a living sacrifice, holy, acceptable unto God, which is your reasonable service.

And be not conformed to this world: but be ye transformed by the renewing of your mind, that ye may prove what is that good, and acceptable, and perfect, will of God. ~

Romans 12:1-2

Hair Care
*Maintenance and Maintain

As women our hair is very important to us. Hair is definitely a crown to a woman of God. Modest hair styles are not only elegant but befitting of a woman of God. Women should see that maintaining the up keep of their hair as an investment. Beauty is an investment. Having a hairstylist is also considered a great investment. Be sure to wash and care for your particular hair texture as much as needed if you are currently unable to afford hair appointments and or your own personal hairstylist. Yes, it's Godly to take good care of yourself as well as your hair. Your hair makes a statement about who you are.

Of course, we all know that certain illnesses and diseases may cause hair to fall out or become brittle. However, whether you are bald or brittle; maintain, take pride in, and groom your head because you are still divinely beautiful either way. Women of God are to be flooded with the light, brilliance, and the overwhelming evidence of God's love in spite of any current illness or disease. Be beautiful while you wait on God's healing. Your appearance speaks of God's great care for you. When people see you, they should see God. When people see you, they should see the glory of God all over you. You are His great masterpiece.

As women of God, we do not wear hair bonnets and pajamas outside the home. In other words, we do not wear hair bonnets and pajamas in public. Hair bonnets and pajamas are to be exclusively reserved for your "at home private life". Stylish hair wraps are beautiful and are made for wearing in public. As women of God, we are to take the initiative to present ourselves as divinely beautiful women of God always. Of course, bad hair days are the inevitable. However, that does not excuse us from doing the best that we can to be presentable. So, with that being said, you are divinely beautiful. Declare it, decree it, and believe it. However, humble yourselves before the Lord, and he will lift you up (James 4:10 NIV). The reward of the humble is promotion by God.

~ I will give thanks to you because I have been so amazingly and miraculously made. Your works are miraculous, and my soul is fully aware of this. ~

Psalm 139:14

Friend Girls
*Be selective

Regals mingle among other regals. Women who desire to become regal in their mindset, behavior, and character are to learn from and watch you (regal) from a distance. You are a leader. Leaders are inspiring. Leaders are worthy of adoration. Leaders are admired. Regals are always leaders. Women of God who are also regal leaders are to minister to others within womanhood from their giftings, talents, and anointing given to them by God. Women of God are to edify, strengthen, and encourage those within womanhood. Women of God are not to be pulled down from their regal status (their God given position). Women of God are not to be involved in cattiness, confusion, drama, maliciousness, vindictiveness, pettiness, and low-life behavior.

As women of God, we know that such behavior is ignited and stirred up by the diabolical one himself, Satan. I advise you not to allow Satan to gain a foothold in your life and relationships. Consider James 4:7 New International Version which declares, "Submit yourselves, then, to God. Resist the devil, and he will flee from you". You do not want him to come in, sabotage, divide, and confuse your relationships with your sisters in Christ. Disallow him. Refuse to engage in such behavior.

Seek and maintain close relationships with women who share your same aspirations: love God, worship God, live for God, prayer, study of the Word, lover of her husband, lover of her family, impactful to her community, involved and engaged in an enjoyable and meaningful life. It is possible for you to have great friendships with other women; knowing that each and every one of you are divinely beautiful. You are God's precious possession/gift. You are not only a gift to and for God but also a gift to the world. Declare it, decree it, believe it. However, humble yourselves before the Lord, and he will lift you up (James 4:10 NIV). The reward of the humble is promotion by God.

~Likewise, teach the older women to be reverent in the way they live, not to be slanderers or addicted to much wine, but to teach what is good. Then they can urge the younger women to love their husbands and children, to be self-controlled and pure, to be busy at home, to be kind, and to be subject to their husbands, so that no one will malign the word of God. ~

Titus 2:3-5

Pretty Girls Fight
*Women are called to be Warriors

The word fight can seem so negative. However, once you become a believer (woman of God) you are enlisted in the army of the Lord (Jesus Christ). Of course, the Lord will see to it that you are trained and equipped through continual fellowship with Him. You are then commanded to fight the good fight of faith. The Bible declares that the weapons of our warfare are not carnal (fleshy) but mighty through God to the pulling down of strong holds (2 Cor 10:4-5). That means believers are not supposed to fight in and through their flesh with physical fist, cuss words, and or any physical contact in regards to spiritual warfare. Remember, Satan and his cohorts are spirits not flesh and blood. You cannot physically fight a spirit. You can cast out a spirit and commanded the spirit to go. Believers do not wrestle with flesh and blood, but against principalities, against powers, against spiritual wickedness in high places. Believers wage warfare against demonic and satanic forces through prayer. Believers are also to stand their ground in the midst of spiritual warfare. Ponder on, "put on the full armor of God [for His precepts are like the splendid armor of a heavily-armed soldier], so that you may be able to successfully stand up against all the schemes *and* the strategies *and* the deceits of the devil".

Your enemies are Satan and his fallen angels (cohorts/subordinates). He (Satan) is your archenemy. The Bible declares that there is and will be enmity (hostility) between woman and Satan (Genesis 3:15). It is clear that there is enmity between Satan and the woman and her offspring; her offspring meaning Jesus Christ (Genesis 3:15). Of course, the woman's offspring which means her natural children are also targets of Satan. All humankind is made in our Lord God's image and likeness. Women of God are to take heart because Satan is already a defeated foe. Women of God are not to fear him. Jesus our Lord won the victory for all humankind. So, when a person being used by Satan or his cohorts comes to discourage you with lies; be vigilant. Ponder on, "Wherefore take unto you the whole armor of God, that ye may be able to withstand in the evil day, and having done all, to stand" (Ephesians 6:13). Remember, be sober [well balanced and self-disciplined], be alert *and* cautious at all times. That enemy of yours, the devil, prowls around like a roaring lion [fiercely hungry], seeking someone to devour (1 Peter 5:8). You are God's great creation and you are divinely beautiful in the natural as well as in the spirit. Declare, decree it, believe it. However, humble yourselves before the Lord, and he will lift you up (James 4:10 NIV). The reward of the humble is promotion by God.

~ So you, my son/my daughter,

be strong [constantly

strengthened] *and* empowered in

the grace that is [to be found

only] in Christ Jesus. ~

2 Timothy 2:1

Mental Health
*What you think on Matters

Your mind is a terrible thing to waste. Most have heard the above statement quoted before. In fact, it's true. All believers should know that one place where Satan attacks is the mind. The battlefield of your life starts and is fought in your mind. As women of God, it is just as important for you to guard your mind (your thought life). Your mind and head are so important God tells you to put on the whole armor of God which includes the helmet of salvation. When women of God put on the helmet of salvation they are able to withstand the attacks coming against their mind through Satan. Thoughts govern actions. As women of God, you should desire to not lose your witness as God's authentic and true vessel. The helmet of salvation is used to protect the brain which is the command station for the rest of the body. If your head becomes badly damaged, the rest of the armor would be of little use.

As believers and women of God we are charged to think on "whatsoever things are true, whatsoever things are honest, whatsoever things are just, whatsoever things are pure, whatsoever things are lovely, whatsoever things are of good report; if there be any virtue, and if there be any praise, think on these things" (Philippians 4:8). Your will, thoughts, and emotions are directly tied to your mental health. As believers, Satan tries his hardest to attack, steal, kill, and destroy us but the secret is that he's already defeated. Satan is counting on you to be ignorant to the fact that he is already a defeated foe (a person who feels enmity, hatred, or malice toward another; enemy, military enemy, hostile enemy). Do not believe the lies of Satan. Be aware of how Satan plays on and attacks the seat of your heart (mind) through your will, thoughts, and emotions.

You are divinely beautiful, fearfully and wonderfully made. Declare it, decree it, and believe it. However, humble yourselves before the Lord, and he will lift you up (James 4:10 NIV). The reward of the humble is promotion by God.

~Humble yourselves [with an attitude of repentance and insignificance] in the presence of the Lord, and He will exalt you [He will lift you up, He will give you purpose]. ~

James 4:10

Physical Health
Your Body is the Temple of Holy Spirit

No matter your body type you are divinely beautiful. We live in a culture where "body shaming" is prevalent. Remember, God never shames you; His Spirit convicts you of wrong doing (sin). In this case, conviction means to convince of an error or sinfulness. For example, gluttony is a habitual greed, over-indulgence, over-consumption, and excessive eating. Gluttony is sin. God is more concerned about your spiritual self vs. your physical self. For example, He desires for your spiritual heart to be right towards Him vs. putting a lot of concentration on your physical heart (a muscular organ). Of course, He desires for you to take care of your temple (body) and heart (a muscular organ) with adequate rest, appropriate consumption of fats and sodium, appropriate consumption of food, and etc. However, when your heart is right towards food you seek to please God by avoiding gluttony.

Food should not be an emotional comfort, emotional support, or crutch. Food should not be used to fill voids. God desires to be your emotional support. He is the healer and possessor of your soul. Ponder on, "He heals the brokenhearted and binds up their wounds" (Psalm 147:3). Also consider, "Come to me, all you who are weary and burdened, and I will give you rest. Take my yoke upon you and learn from me, for I am gentle and humble in heart, and you will find rest for your souls (Matthew 11:28-29).

God desires to be enough for you; to fill any voids. Filling the voids starts with faith in Jesus Christ (Lord God). Growing more and more in love with Jesus will continue to fill any voids that you may have. Remember, as mentioned in Chapter 6 ("Pretty Girls Fight"), be vigilant of your mind (heart), will, thoughts, and emotions. Your mind (heart), will, thoughts, and emotions are to align with Jesus Christ's mind concerning you.

You do not have to be a size two to be healthy. Being a size twenty-two does not mean that you're unhealthy. Genetics and food both play significant roles when factoring in your body type. Knowing who you are in Christ, your fashion, your skin care, your mental health, being able to fight the good fight of faith, and your physical health makes you divinely beautiful. Declare it, decree it, believe it, and behave like it. However, humble yourselves before the Lord, and he will lift you up (James 4:10 NIV). The reward of the humble is promotion by God.

~ Above all else, guard your heart, for everything you do flows from it. ~

Proverbs 4:23

Men
*Men are Your Brothers in Christ

In the kingdom of God, men are your brothers in Christ Jesus. As a woman of God, you must be upfront and pure when dealing with your brothers in Christ. You are precious to God. Your brothers are also precious to God. Dating in the kingdom is different from the way the secular world (unbelievers, sinners, and ungodly) date. Courtship should be the man's objective concerning you. In others words, a Godly man should be attempting to woo you. Woo you with the end results being marriage. To woo, in this context, is to gain the love of someone. Especially with the hopes of marrying that person. Remember, you are the prize. You are the great and valuable possession. Your price is far above rubies. Your job is not to be a silly woman. Silly, in this context, means "morally weak and spiritual dwarfed". Consider this, "They are the kind who worm their way into homes and gain control over gullible women, who are loaded down with sins and are swayed by all kinds of evil desires," (2 Timothy 3:6). Also, think on this, "But I tell you that anyone who looks at a woman lustfully has already committed adultery with her in his heart" (Matthew 5:28).

Depending on where you are in your walk with God, you should be proactively growing out of silliness (your silly days are behind you). You have been redeemed and washed from your transgression by the blood of Jesus Christ. Rest assured your sins are forgiven and forgotten. Men have been called to headship, protectors, priest, kings, messiahs, and providers of their wives and homes. Men are to love their wives with a sacrificial love: loving their wives like Christ loved the church and gave himself up for her. Ponder on, "Husbands, love your wives [seek the highest good for her and surround her with a caring, unselfish love], just as Christ also loved the church and gave Himself up for her," (Ephesians 5:25). Your husband even before he becomes your husband should express the above love towards you.

Wife, woman of God, you are divinely beautiful. Declare it, decree it, believe it. However, humble yourselves before the Lord, and he will lift you up (James 4:10 NIV). The reward of the humble is promotion by God.

~She brings him good, not harm,

all the days of her life. ~

Proverbs 31:12

Salvation Awaits You!

What to do when pursing salvation? You will find the answer to this question in Romans Chapter 10. Romans 10:9-13 Amplified Bible (AMP) because if you acknowledge and confess with your mouth that Jesus is Lord [recognizing His power, authority, and majesty as God], and believe in your heart that God raised Him from the dead, you will be saved. For with the heart a person believes [in Christ as Savior] resulting in his justification [that is, being made righteous— being freed of the guilt of sin and made acceptable to God]; and with the mouth he acknowledges and confesses [his faith openly], resulting in and confirming [his] salvation. For the Scripture says, "Whoever believes in Him [whoever adheres to, trusts in, and relies on Him] will not be disappointed [in his expectations]." For there is no distinction between Jew and Gentile; for the same Lord is Lord over all [of us], and [He is] abounding in riches (blessings) for all who call on Him [in faith and prayer]. For "whoever calls on the name of the Lord [in prayer] will be saved."

About the Author

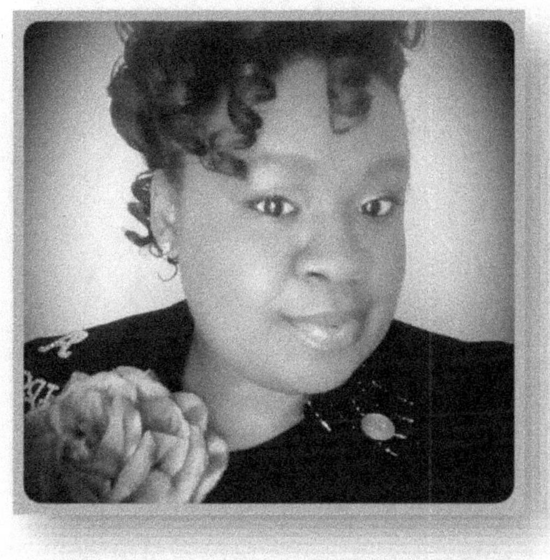

Ashley M. Black

Ashley, a South Carolina resident, holds an Associate Degree in Medical Administration and has
obtained three additional healthcare certifications, and for the last eleven years, has served in healthcare.

Ashley is passionate about sharing the Word of God. She answered the call of ministry in 2013. As a joint heir with Jesus Christ she operates in the Gifts of the Spirit; Word of Knowledge, Word of Wisdom, Prophecy, and in the Gift of Helps. God continues to elevate Ashley from level to level, and from glory to glory. Ashley enjoys raising her son, traveling, and serving the Lord.

References

https://www.biblegateway.com/
https://www.gotquestions.org/
https://biblehub.com/